THE NO-NONSENSE GUIDE TO

a healthy
back

G000161807

THE NO-NONSENSE GUIDE TO

a healthy back

Garry Trainer & Tania Alexander

FOREWORD BY
Dr Hilary Jones

FINGERTIPS
press

"I'd like to dedicate this book
to Victoria, Luke, Max and
all my family in New Zealand."

Garry Trainer

"To Stuart, Alex and Anoushka
with all my love."

Tania Alexander

Fingertips Press Ltd
140 Harley Street
London W1N 1AH

Published by Fingertips Press, 1999.
© Garry Trainer and Tania Alexander

Garry Trainer and Tania Alexander assert the moral right to be
identified as the authors of this work.

A catalogue record for this book is available from the The British Library.

ISBN: 0-233-99762-8

Illustrations: Conny Jude
Design: Keith Hodgson

Production: Portell Productions, London
Reproduction: IGS Ltd., Radstock, Bath
Distributed by André Deutsch Ltd.
Printed and bound in Great Britain by Cromwell Press, Trowbridge, Wilts

NB: The content of this book is designed to complement rather than
replace the advice of your GP or physical therapist. If you experience pain
or strain when following the guidelines or doing any of the exercises in
this book, seek medical advice.

About The Authors

"If anyone knows how the back works it's Garry Trainer"
– Dr Hilary Jones

GARRY TRAINER DO BAc is a renowned osteopath and acupuncturist who combines both these skills to assess and treat back pain. Originally from New Zealand, Garry was a budding sportsman when a serious back injury struck at the age of 17. After three months in hospital and 18 months of drugs and conventional medical treatment, Garry felt as though the bottom had fallen out of his world. Gone were the days of surfing and playing rugby. He was also unable to continue his job as a nurse, as lifting anyone was impossible.

Garry came to England in 1979 to look for any other possibilities of treating his chronic condition. He was recommended acupuncture and was so impressed by the results that he subsequently trained as an acupuncturist (1983) at the London School of Chinese Medicine and then as a osteopath (1985) at the Andrew Stills College. Today, he lives in London with his wife and two children, running a successful practice in Harley Street.

TANIA ALEXANDER is a freelance journalist, specialising in health and fitness. A YMCA fitness instructor and keen sportswoman, she writes for many national publications including The Sunday Times for which she writes a weekly consumer column on health and fitness products. She is fitness consultant to GQ Active, and the author of five books. She lives in London with her husband and two children.

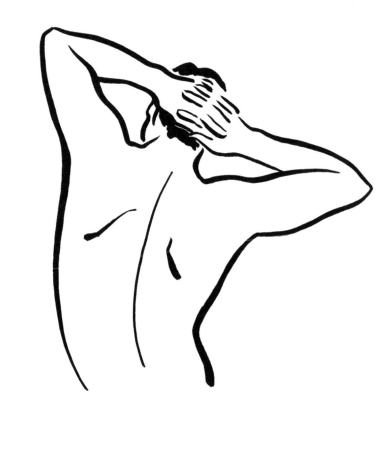

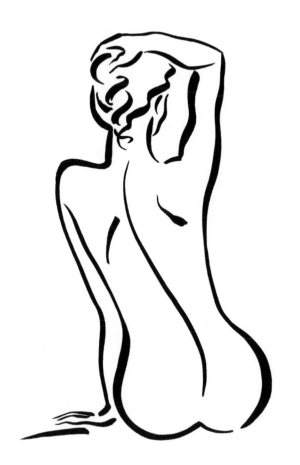

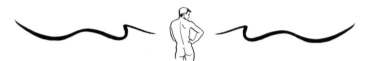

Contents

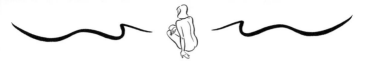

Contents

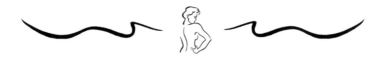

I first met Garry when I was doing a TV programme on back pain with him in 1995. What he said immediately made sense to me from a medical point of view. At the time I was doing a lot of rowing and playing squash. My back was playing up and I was eternally grateful when Garry offered to manipulate it and immediately cleared the problem up.

I'm a firm believer in osteopathy. In the hands of a skilled practitioner like Garry, I truly believe that for many types of back pain, osteopathy is a better line of treatment than conventional medicine.

It's always a good idea to see your GP when you have any sort of medical problem. The main reason for doing this with back pain is so

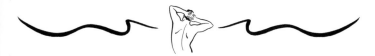

that they can rule out the possibility of any other underlying illness. Sadly the modern GP is so pressed for time that you may not even be examined fully or receive a proper diagnosis.

GPs know that about ninety per cent of people with back pain will get better of their own accord in six weeks, so it is tempting just to send someone off with a prescription for tablets. Unfortunately, this approach could lead to chronic back problems.

Many GPs, myself included, have taken some training in osteopathy. I know from experience that osteopathy can work in a high proportion of cases without taking drugs. There have many occasions when a quick tweak of the spine has proved very effective.

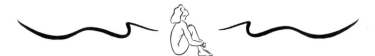

FOREWORD

Most GPs are more than happy to refer you on to an osteopath. A common myth is that osteopaths just deal with back problems. They actually deal with the body as a whole and can sort out all kinds of mechanical problems in the body that lead to other symptoms such as headaches, dizziness, neuralgia, and numbness of limbs.

I'd recommend that people go to an osteopath every year for a check up, just as they'd go to an optician or dentist.

Unfortunately having a strong back isn't second nature. We tend to take the back for granted but when it malfunctions it can turn your life into a misery.

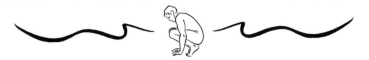

FOREWORD

This is a wonderful little book for getting the facts across and showing people how the simplest actions, like getting out of the car properly or sitting well at a desk, can help prevent problems. Armed with this book, you should be able to make easy positive changes that will enable you to keep your back healthy for life.

Hilary Jones

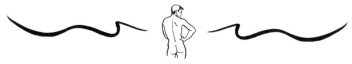

HOW THIS BOOK WORKS

Back pain is a part of modern life. Sixty per cent of adults suffer from back problems. That means even if hasn't happened to you yet, the chances are it will. When it does happen, it can feel that your whole life is tipped upside down. All the little things you took for granted suddenly become an obstacle. Even physically getting out of bed can be a problem.

There are lots of back books on the market. These give a wealth of information about all sorts of different back injuries and how they are treated. Unfortunately, many of them can leave you feeling bombarded with information and even more panicky about what's going on.

This book is designed to give the essential core information about the back and back pain. There is a wealth of information on back pain and how to alleviate it. There are also lots of tips for the lucky minority

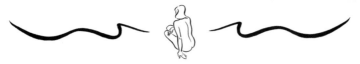

who don't suffer from back pain and want to ensure that they stay in this healthy minority.

The book is full of vital information. It aims to tell you just enough to improve your life without bewildering you.

Of course, no book is a substitute for going to see a doctor or back specialist, so if you still feel worried or confused you should always consult a professional. If you are having treatment, this book works well in conjunction with it.

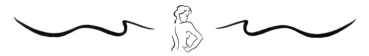

YOU'RE NOT ALONE...

- Back pain keeps 310,000 people away from work every day of the year.

- Each year 22 million people in the UK suffer from some sort of back pain.

- 120 million working days are lost every year in the UK because of back pain.

- Back pain is becoming more prevalent among the 16-24 year age group.

- Back injury is the main reason for people taking long-term sick leave.

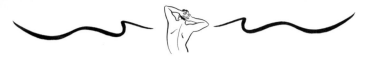

You're not alone...

- 80 per cent of school children carry too much weight in badly designed school bags, often slung over one shoulder, which places considerable strain on young backs. This can cause problems in later life.

- 30 per cent of adults become chronic sufferers.

- Less than 10% of back pain investigations result in surgery.

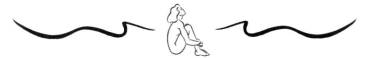

SOD'S LAW BACK PAIN

Stop beating yourself up. It's not always your fault you've got back pain. A common reaction to injuring one's back is "What have I done?" Unfortunately, it's often what we call "Sod's Law Back Pain". You probably didn't do anything dramatic at all. It may well have been an accumulation of stresses. It's often down to simply making the wrong movement at the wrong time. Perhaps you sneezed or coughed or simply moved awkwardly.

The very fact that we move, like all mechanical structures, means we have to expect mechanical problems at some time. Unfortunately, you have more chance of getting back pain than not. But don't worry, help is at hand.

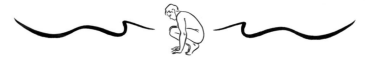

SOD'S LAW BACK PAIN

Ten Common Causes

1. Doing something you're not used to.

2. Lack of exercise.

3. Sitting or standing for prolonged periods.

4. Sleeping awkwardly.

5. Heavy lifting.

6. Pregnancy.

7. Coughing or sneezing.

8. Repetitive movements.

9. Driving.

10. Getting older.

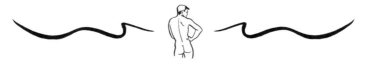

THE BACK DEMYSTIFIED

There is something very mystical about the spine. It is the central supporting system of your body. When something goes wrong with the spine, the whole of your being is affected.

This book is not designed to be a medical textbook. Instead, it aims to give you short, concise information about how the back works and what you can do to keep it healthy and mobile.

The spine is designed to move in six directions - forwards, backwards, laterally (ie side bends) and rotationally (ie twisting round). It is made up of a graceful column of bones called vertebrae, plus the sacrum and coccyx at the base. The spine is more substantial than many people imagine - it's actually deep set

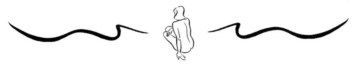

and takes up about half of the body's diameter.

The front inner side of the spine is a smooth S-shaped curve. The back side comprises the individual spines of the vertebrae which you can feel through the skin. Each vertebra moves with the vertibrae above and below it. When these normally mobile joints get stuck problems arise. This sort of back pain is the most common and also one of the easiest to treat.

In between each vertebra is a disc which acts as a shock absorber and nerve roots that feed nerve supply to the whole body.

The spine also acts as casing to protect the vital and fragile spinal cord, part of the central nervous system, which runs down the inside of the spinal column from the base of the brain.

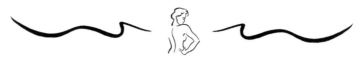

MUSCLES AND NERVES

B ack pain can arise from problems in various spinal structures. Here are two of the most common.

Muscular Pain

SYMPTOMS: Tends to feel worse in the morning and then eases off with movement and as the day progresses.

Muscular pain is the most common type of back pain. A hot bath when you wake up can work wonders. Muscular back pain should always be treated with heat rather than ice unless the muscle is actually torn. Exercising is usually good for this type of back pain, particularly stretching.

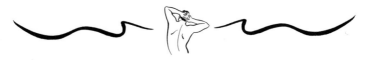

MUSCLES AND NERVES

Nerve Pain

SYMPTOMS: Feels fine while you're resting. You probably feel good first thing in the morning but as the day goes by, the pain gets worse.

Exercise will aggravate this type of back pain, so avoid it. Ice treatments work best - an ice pack at the end of the day is useful. Nerves are much more sensitive structures than muscles, so it would be worthwhile seeing a specialist. Once the pressure is released from the nerve, the pain should be alleviated.

Other causes of pain

Other structures that cause pain are: disc (see page 26), ligament, bone, tendon or capsule. Sometimes x-rays, scans, blood tests and other procedures are necessary to establish an accurate diagnosis.

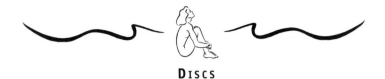

DISCS

The discs are the shock absorbers between the vertebrae. A disk is fairly robust as its gel-like nucleus allows it to change shape according to the pressure put upon it.

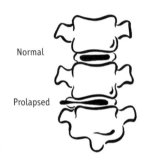

Normal

Prolapsed

If a disc, however, is overloaded it can rupture and cause extreme pain. The most common way to injure a disc is through a twisting action or by lifting a heavy object awkwardly. The disc is normally injured while you are bending forward. If the injury is severe, the disc fluid will start to seep out and may cause compression of the spinal cord, the ligaments, or the nerve roots, which is extremely painful.

There is actually no such thing as a "slipped disc" (although the

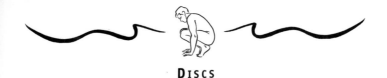

DISCS

fluid within it is slipping out). This is actually referring to a prolapsed disc which is when the disc starts to bulge and protrude. Prolapsed discs are often the result of a violent injury, for example in a contact sport such as rugby.

Discs degenerate with age which is why middle-aged people are susceptible to problems. If you have severe back pain that is not starting to get better after three days of rest (see page 28), it may be a disc problem, particularly if the pain is getting much worse. A classic disc sign is when the real pain comes on 24 hours after the initial twinge.

Disc problems are best treated with lots of rest and passive treatments such as acupuncture for pain relief. If the disc is ruptured and putting pressure on the spinal cord, surgery may be needed. Less than 10 per cent of back injuries actually result in surgery.

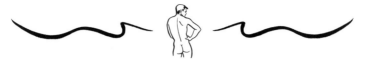

WHAT TO DO IF BACK PAIN STRIKES

If your back gives out, it can be terrifying not knowing what to do, particularly if this is the first time this has happened. Don't panic! In most cases, the back problem will sort itself out providing you rest. Only 20 per cent of back injuries continue to be problematic after two to three days of rest.

FIRST 24 HOURS

- Lie flat on your back, regardless of the type of back pain. Ideally, this should be on a firm surface.

- Try to rest like this for the first 24 hours. Keep everything you need close at hand.

- Don't apply heat in the first 24 hours. Instead, ice the injured area (see page 33).

- Pain killers such as aspirin can be helpful at this stage (see page 30).

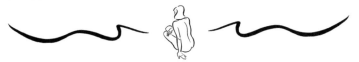

What to do if Back Pain Strikes

DAY 2

Your back may start to feel more bruised than painful. This is a good sign that it's starting to heal. Take it easy. Try to potter around to aid other unaffected areas.

DAY 3

This is D-Day as regards the seriousness of the problem. If the intensity of the symptoms is decreasing, it's very likely that your back is self-regulating itself and there should be no need to see a specialist. If, however, the pain feels worse or you can detect that it's moved (referral symptoms) to the limbs, you should contact an osteopath or similar specialist immediately.

If you are on the road to recovery and you now have an ache rather than a pain, treat with heat rather than ice.

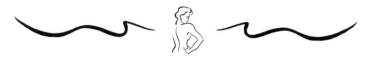

DRUGS

Drugs are very effective at pain relief although they sometimes carry side effects and ideally shouldn't be used long-term.

The most common drugs prescribed for back pain are anti-inflammatory drugs (containing aspirin) but these can sometimes have an adverse reaction on the stomach lining.

Always follow the dose that your GP prescribes and make sure you have eaten something or drunk a glass of milk to line the stomach before taking them.

Muscle relaxants are also commonly prescribed. These help reduce muscle spasm but may make you feel drowsy.

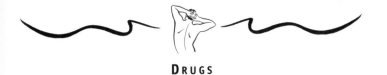

DRUGS

When using drugs, take care not to be over-confident about your progress. You may no longer have the warning signals from pain which prevent you from injuring yourself further.

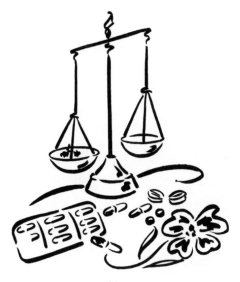

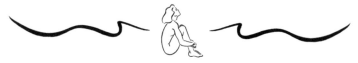

HEAT OR ICE?

When muscles go into spasm because of injury, both heat and ice can be used to desensitize the nerve endings. Different types of back pain respond to different temperatures.

Muscular symptoms usually respond best to heat. If it's an acute muscle strain, or if there's inflammation or swelling, use ice.

To use heat, place a hot water bottle against the most painful part of your back. Alternatively, if the pain is not too severe, soaking in a hot bath may help but you don't want to get yourself in a situation where you get struck by severe pain when you try to get out again.

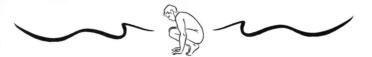

HEAT OR ICE?

If the pain is caused by a nerve being compressed, ice is better.
Place something cold, such as a bag of frozen peas or a can of cold
beer, wrapped in a thin cloth, against the sore area for 10 minutes.
Repeat every 2 hours.

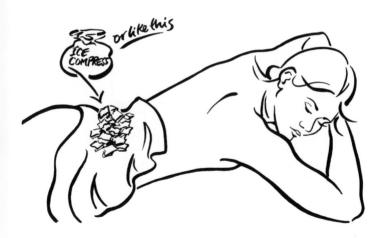

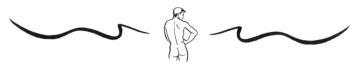

MASSAGE

"Massage is the mother of all therapies".

Massage is a powerful tool that anyone can use. You don't need to be a skilled practitioner. Whether you are suffering from back pain or

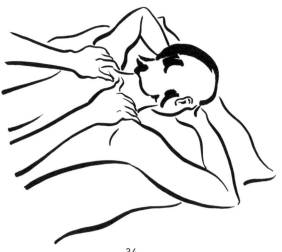

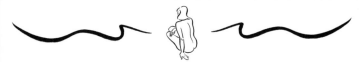

MASSAGE

not, a daily shoulder massage does wonders to relieve tension and relax the back. Strike a deal with your partner that you'll both spend a few minutes each day massaging each other's shoulders.

When it's your turn as masseur, close your eyes and allow your fingers to lead you to the points of tension. Also ask your partner for feedback to direct you to the bits that hurt. When you find a tender area, apply gently pressure there for a few seconds, then release, kneading with thumbs and fingers.

Although it's not quite as enjoyable, you can also massage yourself by squeezing the tops of your shoulders with your fingers or massaging down the sides of your neck with both hands.

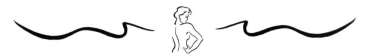

TREATMENT ~ YOUR GP

FACT: Back pain costs the NHS £480 million per year.

The first person you will probably see when you injure your back, is your GP. This is a very good starting point as it can rule out any other medical causes. You will be asked to describe your back pain.

The doctor will give you a thorough physical examination and should be able to make a preliminary diagnosis. You will be probably be recommended bed rest and prescribed pain- killers, anti-inflammatory drugs and muscle relaxants.

If the problem doesn't clear up, the doctor will recommend you to a physical therapist.

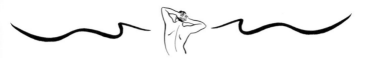

TREATMENT ~ OTHER APPROACHES

Four Approaches To Treatment

Manipulative therapies are very useful in the treatment of back pain because the majority of back pain is mechanical in origin. They work by lubricating the joints' surfaces which restores mobility. Manipulative therapy is an age-old technique. Practitioners used to be referred to as "Bone Setters."

All physical therapies incorporate soft tissue massage and mobilisation of joints and associated structures. Manipulative therapies do this as well as applying a short sharp thrust so that the stretch goes through to the underlying joint.

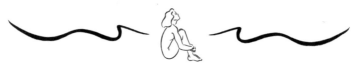

TREATMENT ~ OSTEOPATHY

"In the hands of a skilled practitioner, I truly believe that for many types of back pain, osteopathy is a better line of treatment than conventional medicine," – Dr Hilary Jones.

Osteopathy was founded in 1874 by the American Andrew Taylor Still. It is a system of manual treatment to the spine and other parts of the body. Osteopathy looks at back pain in relation to the whole spine, pelvis, lower limbs and muscle imbalance. Osteopaths spend a minimum of four years training in anatomy, physiology, biomechanics, biochemistry, disease processes and clinical examination and treatment of muscular and skeletal disorders.

The aim of osteopathy is to correct problems in the body frame, making it easier for the body to function normally and reducing the

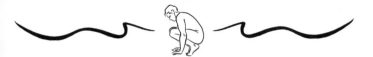

TREATMENT ~ OSTEOPATHY

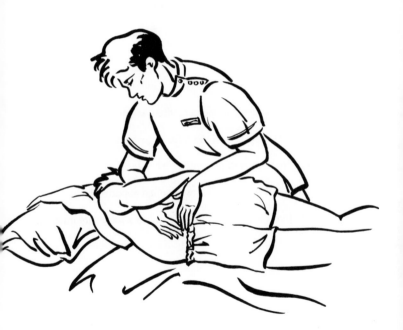

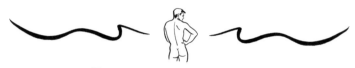

chance of problems occurring in the future. An osteopath often stretches the soft tissues around the joint to bring back the total range of movement. An osteopath may well give advice on diet, something that most conventional doctors might not link to back pain. An osteopath may also advise on posture, lifestyle and stress.

Osteopathy and medicine have a lot in common. They use scientific knowledge of anatomy and physiology. They both use clinical methods of investigation. An osteopath knows enough about pathology to recognise conditions that should be referred to a medically qualified practitioner.

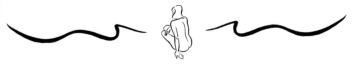

TREATMENT ~ CHIROPRACTIC

The first chiropractic treatment was given by American Daniel David Palmer in 1895. In 1896 he was jailed for practising without a licence. Today thousands of people, particularly back pain sufferers, are helped by this manipulative technique.

The name comes from classic Greek - "chieri" (meaning hand) and "praktikos" (meaning performed). Chiropractors specialise in the diagnosis, treatment and prevention of biomechanical disorders of the musculo-skeletal system, particularly those involving the spine and their effects on the nervous system.

Like osteopathy, chiropractic is very successful in treating back pain. It consists of a wide range of specific manual techniques designed to improve the function of joints, relieve pain and muscle spasm and irritation to the nervous system.

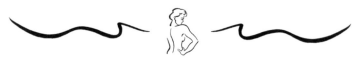

TREATMENT ~ CHIROPRACTIC

Chiropractic treatment is not only for back pain. It also works well for neck pain, arm and leg pain, headaches and many other joint and muscular disorders.

Differences Between Osteopathy And Chiropractic

The differences between osteopathy and chiropractic are slight. Even osteopaths and chiropractors are hard-pressed to explain the differences. As a general rule, chiropractors use more x-rays, particularly for diagnosis and to rule out any underlying problem.

Osteopaths are more cautious to use x-rays, often believing that the information obtained is minimal compared to the risk of radiation.

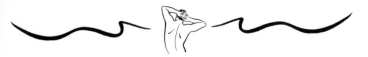

TREATMENT ~ CHIROPRACTIC

What's the crack?

Techniques of treatment between practitioners varies greatly but will

involve gentle manipulation and soft tissue work.

Don't be alarmed if you hear clicks or cracking sounds as the joint

surfaces are moved apart. This is quite normal and won't hurt.

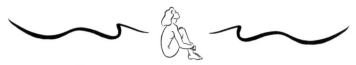

TREATMENT ~ PHYSIOTHERAPIST

Doctors often refer patients to physiotherapists as they both share a medical background. Physiotherapy is available on the NHS.

The physiotherapist will observe the way you walk, stand, sit and bend to assess your condition, diagnose the problem and help you understand what's wrong.

The physiotherapist will work with you to develop an effective treatment plan that takes into account your lifestyle, leisure activities and general health. This will include advice on how you can help yourself such as exercises that you can do between treatment sessions.

Since physiotherapists work primarily with their hands, he or she may be able to treat the back problem by using manipulation and massage.

An infra-red lamp is often used to provide heat which helps the

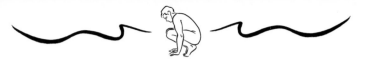

TREATMENT ~ PHYSIOTHERAPIST

muscles to relax. Physiotherapists also use various electrical treatments which stimulate the deeper tissues to encourage drainage and the dispersal of inflammatory waste products and relieve pain.

In general, physiotherapy is fantastic for restoring muscle function after injury or surgery. It also helps to reduce the likelihood of problems recurring.

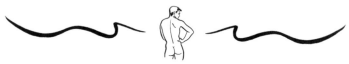

TREATMENT ~ ACUPUNCTURE

FACT: The principle of all physical therapy is to improve the blood supply to the affected area.

Acupuncture is very useful for helping back problems as it's a drug-free way to relieve pain. This ancient method of Chinese medicine relaxes the nervous system by controlling central pain pathways. It also promotes the release of the body's own pain relieving hormones - endorphins. Endorphins have almost the same chemical structure as morphine.

Traditional acupuncture has been used in China as a main form of medicine for thousands of years. The Chinese believe that good health is to be regarded as a state of energy balance within the body. The aim of Chinese medicine is to correct any imbalance in these forces, since

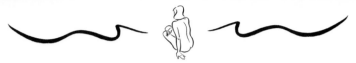

this is the cause of disharmony or disease, and to allow the body's natural healing mechanisms to do the rest.

Today there is a more scientific understanding of how and why acupuncture works and it has been proven to be particularly useful for alleviating pain. It is also surprisingly relaxing. The release of endorphins can now be scientifically measured by taking a sample of spinal fluid before and after treatment.

You don't have to believe in Chinese medicine to understand how acupuncture works. When a fine needle or any foreign body is inserted into the skin, it stimulate the body's defence system to send extra blood to help in whatever way is required. This is an ideal reaction when treating back pain, as the extra blood supply helps reduce muscular spasm, pain and inflammation.

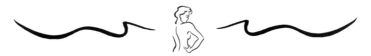

TREATMENT ~ ACUPUNCTURE

Disposable needles are more commonly used to prevent cross-infection. The insertion of fine needles is usually painless. It sometimes produces a mild stinging sensation for a second or two. Once the needles are in place they are left for about 15 minutes. Usually the acupuncturist will twiddle the needles to adjust the energy flow.

Although you can relieve muscle spasm by other physical therapies such as massage, acupuncture is a more refined way of hitting the exact spot. Results can be quite dramatic.

If you are needle-phobic, there are other ways to stimulate the acupressure points - laser, electrical, heat or finger pressure.

As it's so gentle, acupuncture is an ideal treatment choice for the elderly.

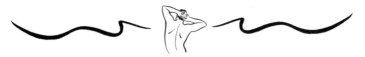

TREATMENT ~ OTHER ALTERNATIVES

There are many alternative therapies which can help alleviate back pain. These may be worth investigating, particularly if you're suffering from chronic pain and want to avoid long-term use of conventional drugs.

HOMEOPATHY is based upon the principle "like cures like". Homeopathic remedies such as Arnica can be prescribed to help all sorts of back conditions.

HERBALISM uses medicines prepared from plants. They can help alter the biochemical imbalances which cause pain and stiffness. For example, white willow bark has the same anti-inflammatory properties as aspirin. Herbal medicines can be taken orally as tablets or as

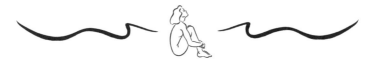

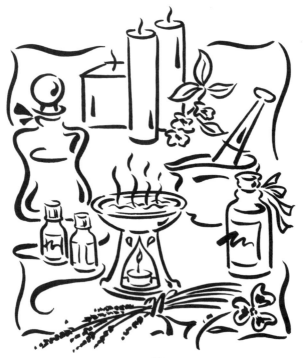

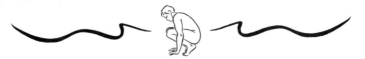

infusions. Dried or fresh herbs may also be added to a hot bath.

AROMATHERAPY uses essential oils, extracted from plants for specific and therapeutic effect. The oils are usually diluted in a carrier oil such as almond oil and then massaged into the skin. They are rapidly absorbed into the bloodstream. Alternatively you can put a few drops in the bath.

You should always go to a qualified practitioner to prescribe a natural remedy for you. Ideally, you should try to find someone who has been referred by a few reliable sources. Good practitioners get good results so their reputation should precede them.

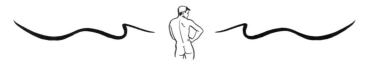

POSTURE

A lot of back pain is simply due to poor posture. If you are a back pain sufferer, it is certainly worth working on your posture in the hope of improving or at least preventing things getting worse.

Posture Test

Check your posture by standing in bare feet with your back to the wall. Slowly press your body back to touch the wall. If you have good posture just your hair, shoulder-blades and bottom should touch the wall. You should be able to place one hand between the wall and your lower back. If you can place a whole fist between your lower back and the wall, or your shoulders touch the wall before your bottom, your pelvis is too far forward and you need to practise the Pelvic Tilt (see page 115). If you feel that one side of your body touches before the

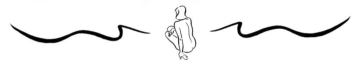

POSTURE

other, you are lop-sided and need to work on levelling your body out with lots of side bends (see page 100 and 104). If your entire body is in contact with the wall, your posture is too rigid - this can lead to fatigue and laboured breathing. It also produces a lot of tension in the neck. You need to soften out.

Postural Techniques

The Alexander Technique (see page 56) is extremely effective at improving posture. Exercise systems such as yoga and Pilates also place much emphasis on correct body alignment.

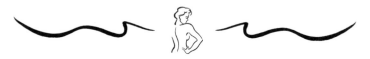

POSTURE ~ YOUR SPINE

The Shape Of Your Spine

Apart from the normal spine (see page 22) there are three other main categories.

Lordosis – often called "sway back" this type of spine hollows out in the lower back.

Kyphosis – this is an exaggerated thoracic curve that results in a hunched back.

Scoliosis – this is curvature of the spine. Instead of being straight, the spine takes an s-shaped curve. Mild cases of scoliosis are very common and can be helped with stretching exercises to straighten out the bend.

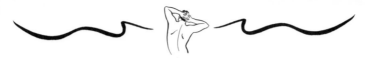

POSTURE ~ YOUR SPINE

Although you can't change the shape of the spine you were born with, improved posture and regular stretching exercises can help rebalance the situation.

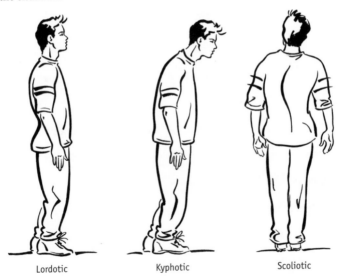

Lordotic   Kyphotic   Scoliotic

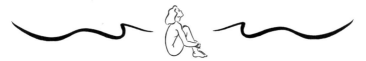

POSTURE ~ THE ALEXANDER TECHNIQUE

The Alexander Technique was devised by an Australian actor called Frederick Matthias Alexander who was born in 1869 in Wynyard, Tasmania. It is a system of re-educating the body so that it is correctly aligned.

The theory is that it can then function as nature intended. With its strong emphasis on posture, it can be a useful way to both treat and prevent back pain.

When you go to see an Alexander Technique practitioner, you will be guided through a series of physical movements that can then be practised on a daily basis.

Although many of these look easy, such as standing up from a chair, when you start to practise them you will realise how much can go wrong even with the simplest of movements.

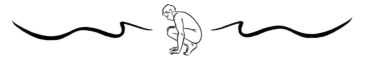

POSTURE ~ THE ALEXANDER TECHNIQUE

You will be taught postures specifically designed for your own posture, which need to be practised regularly. You will probably find you have to undo all the bad postural habits that you have picked up over the years.

In the beginning, the correctly aligned posture may feel unnatural or even uncomfortable, but with practice, these can make a tremendous difference to the health of your back.

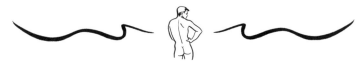

POSTURE ~ STANDING

The human body is designed to be on all fours which distributes the weight evenly throughout the spine. When upright all the weight concentrates on the lower back.

Try to work on improving your posture whenever you are standing. Pull your stomach muscles in (the more you work these, the stronger they will become which not only looks good but helps support your back). Your lower back should be slightly curved but not hollowed out. Keep your shoulders down and your neck long.

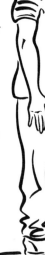

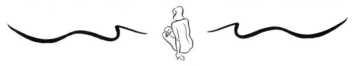

POSTURE ~ STANDING

Standing For Long Periods

This can place the spine under strain. Pelvic tilts are excellent for taking the pressure off the lower spine (see page 115). Elasticated supports (or even a scarf tied round your lower back) can also be helpful. Additional support is temporary and should not be relied on for long periods of time.

Another good way to relieve pressure when standing is to rest one foot on a raised platform (such as a telephone directory), making sure you change legs.

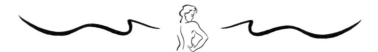

POSTURE ~ INVERSION

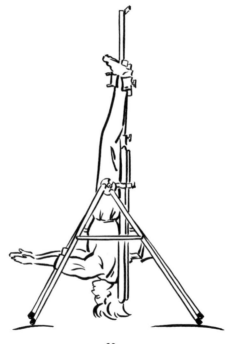

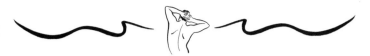

POSTURE ~ INVERSION

Inversion

The fact that human beings are standing upright on two legs causes a lot of pressure on the spine as it means gravity is constantly pressing down and reducing disc space. As there is less space for the nerves they are more easily impinged.

Many people find great relief from inversion, either hanging upside down in anti-gravity boots or in a back swing frame. This can feel very relaxing and allows the vertebrae to pull apart and create more space. Inversion products can be purchased from specialist back shops and sports stores.

Traction is a common technique used in physical therapy, and like inversion it is used to take the pressure off the spine.

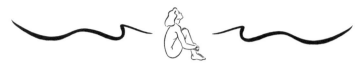

POSTURE ~ SITTING

Sitting for long periods of time can also be bad for the spine. Try to sit upright as much as possible with abdominals pulled in for support. Check that both feet are flat on the floor. Don't worry if you occasionally slouch. This is perfectly normal and won't do you any harm providing you balance it by maintaining good posture for most of the day.

Choosing a chair

If much of your day is spent sitting down, it is worth investing in a decent chair. Check that it has good lumbar support (you can buy lumbar support cushions). Sometimes a rolled up towel will suffice. Ideally the chair should be tilted so that the seat slopes gently downwards, ensuring that your knees are lower than your hips.

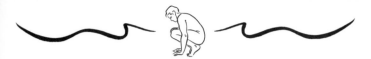

POSTURE ~ SITTING

A wedge cushion can be used to the same effect for a much lower cost.

Sitting at a desk

If you're working at a PC, check that the desk or table is at an appropriate height. If you spend much time looking at paperwork, try to avoid hunching over it. Ideally you should have a stand on the desk so that any

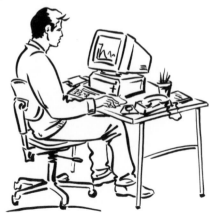

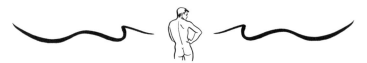

POSTURE ~ SITTING

written matter is at eye level and you don't need to keep looking down or turning round. If your neck starts to feel tense when you're sitting, check that you are not losing correct alignment of the neck by jutting your chin out.

Counterbalance the strain of prolonged sitting by taking an active break every 30 minutes. See page 102 for seated stretches.

Also see BACK PAIN AT WORK (page 68)

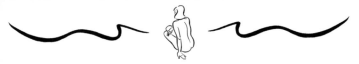

POSTURE ~ LYING DOWN

Lying down flat is often the most comfortable position if you have back pain. In fact, pain can often be alleviated simply by lying on a hard floor for five or ten minutes.

Lying down reduces the pressure on the spine and helps decrease compression. Sometimes it is more comfortable to lie with your knees bent and feet flat on the floor as this takes some of the strain off the lumbar spine.

Try to flatten the small of your back into the floor. Place your hand underneath your lower back to check.

Also see AND SO TO BED (page 72)

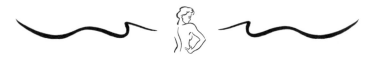

POSTURE ~ LIFTING

The back should not be used like a crane. One of the most common ways to injure your back is through poor lifting technique. It doesn't even have to be a heavy object - you can injure yourself just by bending down awkwardly to pick up a piece of paper.

Lifting Plan

- Always keep your back straight.

- Allow your quadriceps (thigh muscles) to do the work rather than your back.

- Take a wide stable stance and squat

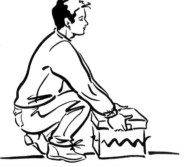

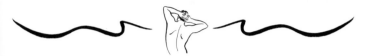

down, keeping your head up, stomach pulled in and back straight.

- You may feel more stable squatting with one foot slightly in front of the other.

- Grasp the object firmly and pull it in close to your body.

- Stand up in one slow smooth movement.

- Keep your head up and push with your legs.

- Maintain close body contact with the object you are lifting. Make sure you're wearing suitable clothing so that you can hold the weight close to you without worrying about messing up your clothes.

- When carrying an object to another location, make sure you've prepared the route by looking out for obstacles such as kids' toys.

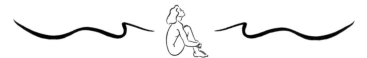

MANAGING BACK PAIN ~ AT WORK

FACTS

- Nearly 200 million working days are lost in the UK due to certified incapacity through back pain.

- The cost to industry in lost production from back pain is at least £6 billion.

T he most hazardous jobs, from a back point of view, are those that involve prolonged periods of sitting (see page 62).

Tips at work

- Maintain good posture at all times. The odd slouch is allowed.

- Check your feet are flat on the floor or on a foot rest.

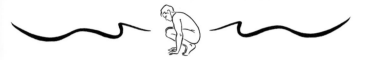

MANAGING BACK PAIN ~ AT WORK

- Don't cross your legs - this restricts circulation and puts your spine out of alignment.

- Keep your forearms in a horizontal position and wrists supported when using a VDU or PC.

- Position the phone on your desk so that it's on the same side that you answer it with. Avoid crooking the phone in between your head and neck. If you're on the phone a lot in the day, a headset is a good idea. If you use a mobile, use a hands free device.

- If you have a sedantary job try to do something active like a brisk walk at lunchtime or a swim or a yoga class after work. The more sedentary your job the more you need to balance this with extra physical activity outside work.

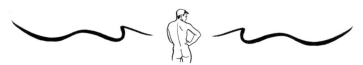

Old-fashioned beds tend to be much kinder on the back as they are much higher and safer to get in and out of.

Mattresses

Soft mattresses do not support the spine sufficiently, encouraging the body to sag. This can place both ligaments and joints under strain. A good mattress should be firm and contour its shape around the bod, but not so hard as to be uncomfortable.

Pillows

Should be supportive to the neck. If you need extra support under the neck, place a small rolled towel in your pillowcase. There are also special support pillows on the market.

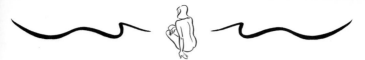

MANAGING BACK PAIN ~ AND SO TO BED

Position

Ideally you should sleep on your back or side. In the former case, slip a
pillow under your calves as this will help reduce the lumbar curve.
When lying on your side, a pillow between your knees creates a more
stable base.

Morning stretch

Like a cat or dog, start the day by waking your spine up gently.
Lie on your back in the middle of the bed hugging your knees for a
few seconds into your chest. Now stretch your arms out to the side.
Keeping your knees bent in, slowly lower to one side so you feel a
stretch up the side of the spine. Hold for 5-10 seconds. Repeat on the
other side.

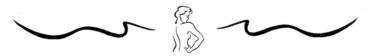

MANAGING BACK PAIN ~ AND SO TO BED

Getting out of bed

1. Lie on your side at the edge of the bed.

2. As you drop your lower limbs onto the floor, push up on to your elbow and then to the upright position using your arm. You may use your other hand to push off the bed for extra leverage.

3. The weight of your legs dropping down will help pull your upper body up with less strain to the back.

Making the bed

Adopt good posture by squatting down to make the bed, keeping spine straight, stomach pulled in and head up. Avoid twisting. Fitted sheets and duvets cause less strain.

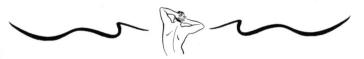

Managing Back Pain ~ And So To Bed

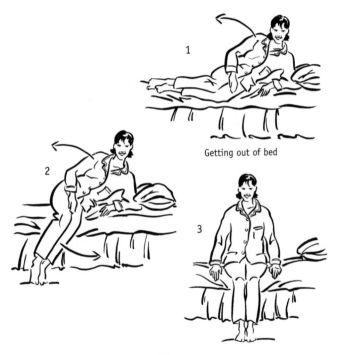

Getting out of bed

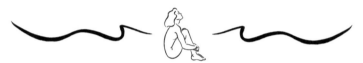

"Not tonight, darling, I have back pain."

Although having sex is not a good idea in the acute phase of back injury, it can be a good technique for mobilising the pelvis. Back pain is often used as an excuse for avoiding sex. In many cases, however, gentle love-making is actually very beneficial for the back. The gentle rhythmic rolling of the pelvis can be very soothing to back pain sufferers. This pelvic thrust motion works well as a mobilising exercise.

Choosing Positions

Choose the position that feels more comfortable for you. If you both have bad backs, it's best to do it from the side. All fours, with the man entering from behind, is a good position for female back sufferers. Just make sure you don't arch your back.

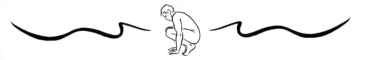

MANAGING BACK PAIN ~ SEX

The man sitting on a chair with his partner on top is good for both of you, regardless of who has the back pain.

Tips

- If you do experience some back pain while making love, don't panic! Just slow down or stop if the pain is severe. This is not a time to break records.

- Start your love-making by massaging each other. This will soothe your back and is wonderful foreplay.

- Experiment with positions and go with what feels most comfortable. Back pain may actually be the best thing that ever happened to your sex life!

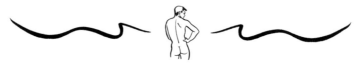

Back pain is very common in pregnancy. There are two main reasons for this. During pregnancy the body produces a hormone called relaxin which softens the ligaments and connective tissues in the body. This allows the usually stable joints of the pelvis to loosen up to enable the baby to be delivered.

The shape of the pregnant woman also puts the spine under stress. The enlarging abdomen and breasts throws the body off balance and often results in an over-curved lower back which can lead to pain and strain.

The good news is that a pregnant woman is very easy to treat for back pain as her body is so mobile and responsive to very gentle manipulation. Physical therapies such as osteopathy and chiropractic are perfectly safe in pregnancy and usually have excellent results.

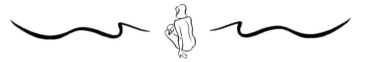

MANAGING BACK PAIN ~ PREGNANCY

Tips

- Try not to gain excess weight. Keep within recommended guidelines (between 11.3-15.9 kgs/ 25-35 lbs).

- Avoid wearing high heels as that will encourage you to arch your back even more.

- Be particularly careful with lifting (see page 66).

- Avoid standing for long periods. Rest one foot on a stool, knees bent for support.

- Tying a scarf or wearing a support belt under your bump can often alleviate back pain.

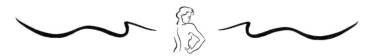

MANAGING BACK PAIN ~ PREGNANCY

Recommended

This is an excellent mobilisation exercise for everyone, but particularly

soothing when you are pregnant. Kneel on all fours with your hands and

knees about shoulder-width apart. Drop your stomach and chest towards

the floor while raising your bottom towards the ceiling (see a). Extend the

neck slightly. Now drop your head and arch your back upwards (see b).

a. Arching the spine

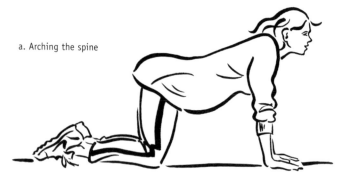

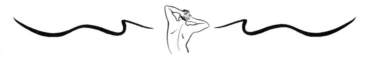

It also feels great if the pregnant woman has someone place a hand on her sacrum (the bottom of the spine) while she's in the neutral all-fours position (see c). Apply gentle pressure here and make small circular motions to help mobilise the pelvis

b. Rounding the spine

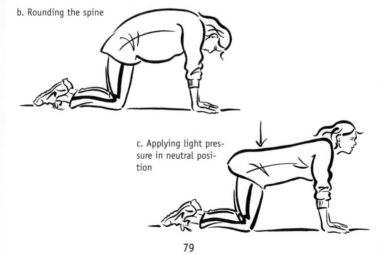

c. Applying light pressure in neutral position

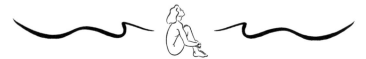

Managing Back Pain ~ Children

Back pain in children is increasing, as their lifestyle becomes more and more sedentary.

- Slouching in front of the TV or playing computer games is not doing your child's health any good. Limit passive pursuits like this to a maximum of two hours a day. Encourage them to strengthen and stretch their muscles through outdoor games.

- Increase the whole family's activity levels by Sunday morning walks or football in the park.

- Walk, or at least walk part of the way, with your child to school. Most children are far too reliant on being ferried everywhere by car.

- Buy your child a rucksack. Research shows that heavy school bags slung over one shoulder are causing back problems in children. Talk to

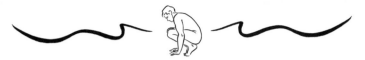

your teacher about the school's seating. Many school chairs are poorly designed. One solution would be to have foam wedges on the chairs to encourage the correct pelvic alignment.

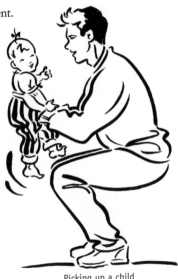

Although you don't have any choice, looking after babies and small children can be hazardous for the back. There are ways you can minimize the stress to the spine.

Picking them up

Always bend from the knees, keeping the weight of the child as close

Picking up a child

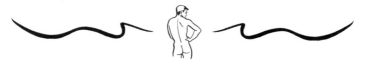

to your body as possible. Never twist round when you're in a bent position as this is the easiest way to damage the back. Remember to keep your head up and use your leg power for leverage.

Carrying infants

Many mothers make the mistake of hitching the infant over one hip which in the long term can cause imbalance and strain. Switch sides regularly.

Tidying up

Squat rather than bend down. If you're tidying up a lot of toys, make sure you kneel or squat rather than stoop.

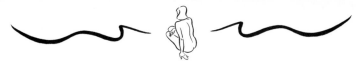

Baby care

Look for a cot that has a drop side and is of a reasonable height so that you don't have to bend over it. If necessary, place blocks or telephone directories underneath it to create the right height.

Check that the pram and push chair are at a comfortable height so you maintain good posture.

When bathing a baby, place the baby bath on a table that is at an appropriate height and don't try to empty all the water in one go without help.

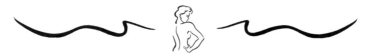

MANAGING BACK PAIN ~ THE ELDERLY

One has to expect wear and tear on the spine, like any other part of the body, with increasing age. As you get older, bones become thinner and more porous. Bony spurs (osteophytes) often grow on the vertebrae, discs start to degenerate and thin and soft tissues lose their flexibility.

Exercise (particularly weight-bearing exercise such as walking) is very important for the elderly. Swimming is a good general exercise that is ideal for fragile bones as it's non-impact. At this time of life, maintaining suppleness and mobility is vital. Daily stretching and mobility routines can make a tremendous difference to well-being. Preventative treatment is recommended. Physiotherapy is excellent for ensuring you keep all your joints mobile.

An elderly person with back pain can also be treated with physical

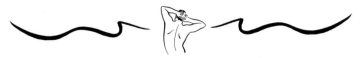

therapies such as osteopathy but this has to be approached very gently using passive techniques rather than high velocity thrusts.

When you're young, you can fall over hard and just get up and carry on. When you're old, falling can be the beginning of the end. Unfortunately, we become more unstable as we grow old therefore it's easier to fall. Elderly people need to work hard at maintaining good postural habits and muscle tone. If there is any time in your life that you need to stay active, it's now.

There are many gadgets on the market designed to make everyday life easier for the elderly and these are worth investigating.

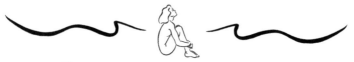

MANAGING BACK PAIN ~ DRIVING

Driving is one of the most common places for back ache to start. The simple reason is that you're in a seated position for a long period of time.

When sitting in the car, concentrate on good posture at all times. Keep the steering wheel as close to you as possible as this will create less strain on the back when you turn the wheel. A good lumbar support in the seat can help. A neck rest is also a good idea.

Take care getting in and out of the car, particularly if the car is low to the ground. Slide your bottom in first with your feet on the pavement. Then slowly swivel round to face forward with your hands on the seat for support.

If you have to put children into the back, it's very useful to have a four door car. If you can't face parting with your sporty two-door

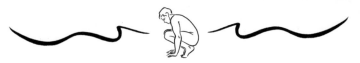

coupe, make sure you climb into the back with them before fiddling about with car seats or rear seat belts.

Never twist round to pick up parcels from the back seat. On long journeys, try to take regular breaks when you can get out of the car and do a small stretch routine.

If you are a chronic back pain sufferer you may want to consider trading in your manual car for an automatic with power steering.

After a long car journey go for a long walk. This is not the time to slump in front of the TV.

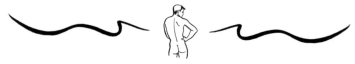

GARDENING

Gardening is very therapeutic. It's also a classic place to injure your back.

TIPS

- Take care when bending down and picking things up. Remember to keep your back straight, knees bent, head up and the load as close to your body as possible.

- Avoid prolonged bending and stooping by kneeling or squatting instead. A gardener's kneeling pad is useful.

- Use long-handled implements whenever possible to avoid unnecessary reaching or bending.

- When sweeping or hoeing, keep to a forward and backwards action. Unless you have very strong stabilising muscles, any sweep-

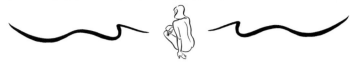

ing motions across the body can put the back at risk.

- When using a lawn mower, use your body weight to help the movement. Look for as light a mower as possible so that you don't have anything too heavy to haul around.

- Watch the wheelbarrow as it's a very unstable design.

- If your back is playing up ask a friend or fitter member of the family to help with the heavy work.

- Take regular breaks from gardening to do some stretches. Stretching outdoors is particularly enjoyable.

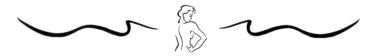

HEALTHY EATING

If you are overweight, you will be placing your back under further strain. The classic beer belly shape throws your body out of alignment and places a strain through your lower back.

Diets don't work which is why the slimming industry is so wealthy as people keep coming back for more. Forget about losing weight instantly. Crash diets result in a decreased metabolic rate (your body simply stores fat as it's scared of being starved). This is why you find that once you start eating normally again, you end up even fatter than you were before the diet.

The only way to lose weight is to re-educate your eating patterns. Keep a food diary, recording everything you eat over a period of five days. Instead of eating less try to substitute some of the more fattening foods (alcohol, cakes, biscuits, pastries, butter, cheese, chocolate, crisps,

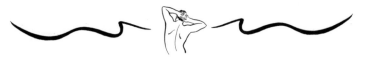

chips, ready- prepared meals and fried foods) with raw fresh foods such as vegetables, fruits and nuts. Although these will taste exceptionally bland at first, once your palate adjusts, you'll be surprised what an energy boost you can get from a couple of bananas or a plate of crudites and nuts.

Don't deny yourself

Denying yourself foods altogether also doesn't work as it turns that food into more of an issue. Allow yourself a couple of days a week (such as the weekend) when you can consume some of the less healthy foods or drinks that you really crave.

If you have arthritis, it is worth seeing a nutritionist who can advise on a special diet to help your condition.

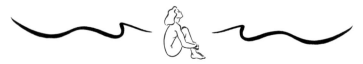

HEALTHY EATING

Healthy Eating Tips

- Increase your intake of water to about two litres a day. Dehydration is often masked as hunger so once you've had a drink, you may lose that urge to have a snack.

- Eat little and often and avoid bingeing.

- Never go shopping on an empty stomach

- Concentrate on the food you eat. Avoid doing anything else such as watching TV, talking or reading while eating as you won't be so aware when you're full.

- If you have a bad eating day, try to expend some of the extra calories through exercise the next day.

Remember, overweight people are not the only ones to suffer back pain but excess weight will make you more susceptible.

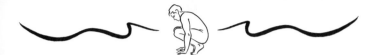

HEALTHY EATING

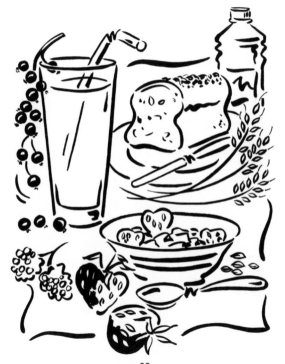

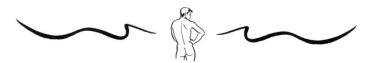

EXERCISE

R egular exercise is important both for alleviating and preventing back pain. A sedentary lifestyle is not doing your health any good and you can't expect your spine to function properly if you're not maintaining its mobility.

The two most important types of exercise from the back's point of view are stretching and strength training. Don't panic! This doesn't mean you have to join your local gym. All back exercises can be done at home and will easily slot into your everyday life. Look for opportunities when you can stretch, such as lying in the bath or sitting at your desk at work.

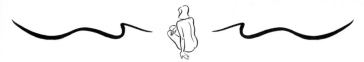

EXERCISE

Tips

Find a time of day to exercise that best suits your lifestyle. If you like a slow leisurely start to the day, begin with some gentle stretches as soon as you get out of bed or even in bed. If you need to slowly unwind at night, do your stretches before you go to bed.

It's best to warm up before doing any exercise as this makes your muscles more pliable and less susceptible to strain. Warm up by walking briskly around the house or just marching on the spot and doing some simple mobility exercises such as arm raises, little knee bends or hip circles. A hot bath before stretching is also a good idea.

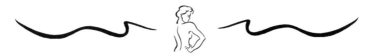

EXERCISE ~ STRETCHING

Stretching is one of the most enjoyable types of exercise and is particularly beneficial for your back as it keeps it mobile and reduces most muscular tension. Watch any animal such as a cat, and you'll see how stretching is an instinctive part of their day.

Aim to stretch every day so it becomes a habit like brushing your teeth. This will only take you a few minutes and you will be amazed how quickly your flexibility improves. After warming up, ease gently into a stretch until you feel a tiny bit of tension. This tension is caused by what is known as the "stretch reflex" - the body's way of protecting itself from injury.

When you try to stretch a muscle, the brain makes the muscle contract in order to prevent it from being over-extended or damaged. The more you try to force the stretch, the stronger the stretch reflex

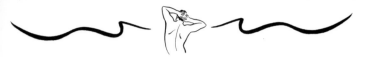

EXERCISE ~ STRETCHING

fires and the more tension and even pain you will feel in the muscle.

When you reach this initial point of tension, hold the stretch quietly until the stretch reflex backs off as it thinks the muscle is out of danger. This takes about 6-10 seconds. Then slowly develop the stretch by gently easing into it until you feel the stretch reflex restraining you again. Continue trying to develop the stretch for up to 30 seconds.

Remember, for back care you need to regularly stretch the back in six directions (forwards, backwards, side to side and twisting round).

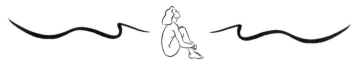

EXERCISE ~ STANDING STRETCHES

The following stretches will take you
through all six required directions in the
standing position.

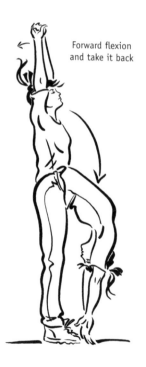

Forward flexion
and take it back

Forward Flexion

Stand with your feet hip width apart,
stomach pulled in, spine long. Reach
up to the ceiling with both hands
without arching your back. Slowly
let your arms reach down towards the
floor, keeping your stomach pulled in.
Don't worry if you can't touch the floor.
Let your head and arms hang.

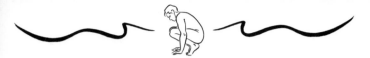

EXERCISE ~ STANDING STRETCHES

If you find it difficult to bend forward, bend your knees.

Take It Back

Stand as above. This time, as you stretch your arms up take them back behind you so that you are hyper-extending your back. Keep your stomach muscles pulled in for support. Don't extend too far.

Side Bends

Stand with your feet hip-width apart (see over page). Place your right hand on right thigh. Pull your stomach in as you take your left arm up and over towards your right side. Imagine there is a sheet of glass in front and behind you to keep you well aligned. Your hips stay pointing forwards throughout. Repeat on other side.

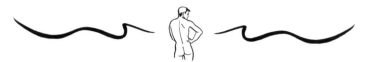

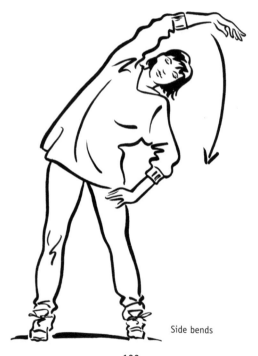

Side bends

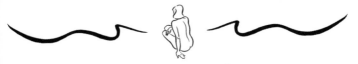

EXERCISE ~ STANDING STRETCHES

The Twist

Stand with a wall about six inches behind you. Slowly twist round to the left, using your arms on the wall for leverage. Try to keep hips facing forwards. Repeat on other side.

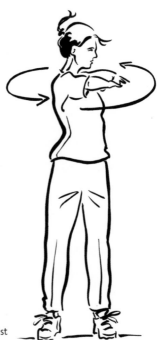

The twist

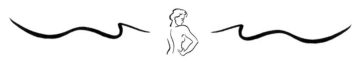

EXERCISE ~ SEATED STRETCHES

A chair is actually a useful tool for stretching. The same six-direction principle applies.

Forward Flexion

Sit tall with your stomach pulled in. Reach up with both arms, taking care not to arch your back. Bend forward so that you rest your chest on your thighs, allowing head and arms to hang loose.

Take It Back

As you take your arms up, extend your neck and upper back backwards. Keep your stomach muscles pulled in.

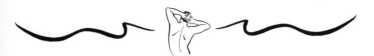

EXERCISE ~ SEATED STRETCHES

Forward flexion
and take it back

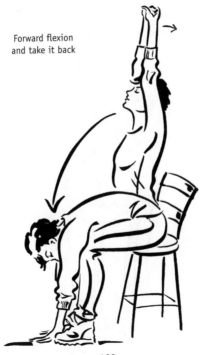

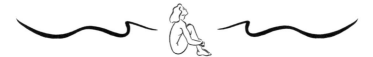

EXERCISE ~ SEATED STRETCHES

Side bends

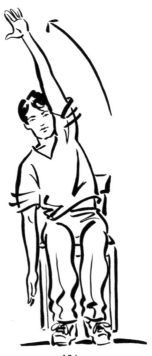

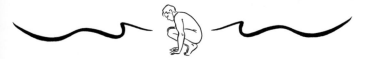

EXERCISE ~ SEATED STRETCHES

Side Bends

As in standing, resting your left hand on your left thigh or by your side as you take your arm over to the right and vice versa.

The Twist

Twist round using the back of the chair for leverage. Keep hips facing forward, abdominals pulled in.

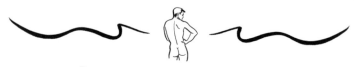

EXERCISE ~ FLOOR STRETCHES

If you have a bad back, doing exercises on the floor gives you the most support and stability. You can also do some of these in the bath or in bed. These movements are an excellent start to any stretching routine and very soothing to the back.

Waking up your spine

The Hug

Lie on your back and hug your knees into your chest. Now gently rock gently from side to side. This is a small movement that feels as though you are massaging your spine – your knees do not drop to the floor.

Rock and Roll

Start in the hug position. Rock forward to an upright seated position

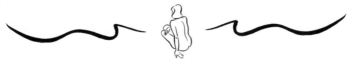

EXERCISE ~ FLOOR STRETCHES

and then roll back, aiming to roll your lower back vertebra by vertebra off the floor. Aim to build up a smooth flowing motion. This is an excellent self-massage and mobility techniques.

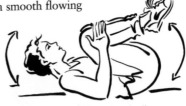

Rock and roll

Forward Flexion

Forward flexion

Sit with your legs stretched out in front of you (this is a good one to do in the bath). Reach up and forward, aiming to touch your toes with your fingertips.

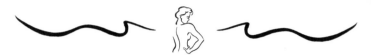

EXERCISE ~ FLOOR STRETCHES

Don't worry if you can't reach at first. This is a good exercise for stretching out the hamstring muscles as well as the back. Tight hamstrings often play a part in back ache.

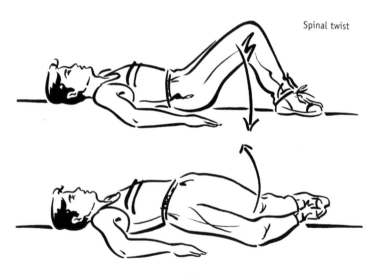

Spinal twist

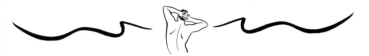

EXERCISE ~ FLOOR STRETCHES

Spinal Twist

Lie on your back. Bend your knees with your feet flat on the floor. Extend your arms out to the sides. Slowly roll your knees over to one side so that you feel a stretch up the side of the back. Return to centre and repeat on other side. To increase the stretch hug your knees into your chest and drop them over to the floor in this position.

Alternative Twist

Sit on the floor with your legs stretched out in front of you. Bend your right leg, foot flat on floor. Place your left elbow on the outside of your right knee. Slowly rotate your body round to the right using your left elbow for leverage. Repeat on other leg.

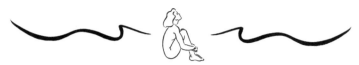

EXERCISE ~ UPPER BODY STRETCHES

The stretches below are good for alleviating tension in the neck, shoulders and upper back. They can be done sitting, standing or kneeling. Take care not to arch your lower back. Start by releasing tension in the shoulders by doing some shoulder rolls in both directions.

Upper Back

Stretch your arms up above you, fingers clasped and palms of hands facing ceiling. Don't arch your back. Take the stretch out to the side for a side stretch.

Neck

Keeping your shoulders down, gently drop your head to the right until

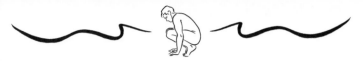

you feel a stretch down the left side of the neck. You can use your right hand for a little extra leverage. Repeat on other side.

Shoulders

Hold your right upper arm with your left hand and pull the right arm over across your body so you feel a stretch in the right shoulder. Repeat on other side.

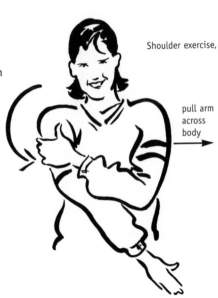

Shoulder exercise,

pull arm across body

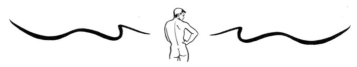

EXERCISE ~ STRENGTH TRAINING

Strength work is best performed every other day as your muscles need a day in between to rest and repair themselves which is all part of the strength- building process. Strong muscles will help protect your back from injury.

Ideally, you should follow a general strength-training programme, targeting all major muscle groups. Most strength-training can be done at home using your own body weight for resistance.

If you want to use weights, you can start with everyday objects such as bottles of water or tins of food. Resistance bands are also an economical alternative to weight sets.

From the back's points of view, you at least need to do regular back and abdominal work. The abdominals are the opposing muscle group to the erector spinae (back muscles). If these are not in

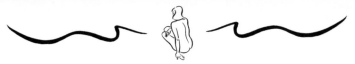

EXERCISE ~ STRENGTH TRAINING

balance, pain and injury can result.

Build up the number of reps slowly. Strength training is all about progression. Don't worry if you can only do one rep to start with. In a couple of months you will be doing 20. The elderly should concentrating on adding repetitions rather than weight.

Always prepare your muscles by stretching the muscles you intend to strengthen.

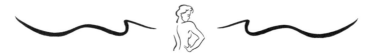

EXERCISE ~ STRENGTHENING THE BACK

Lie on your stomach with your hands by your sides. Raise up and hold the extension for ten seconds. Slowly return to the floor. Rest for five seconds. If you can do this 20 times you have good muscle tone in the lower back. If you can only do five, do six the next time and add one on each session. Remember for best results strength training should be done every other day.

Stop if causing pain.

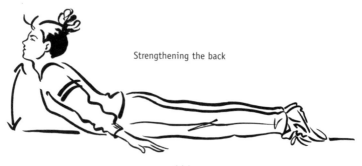

Strengthening the back

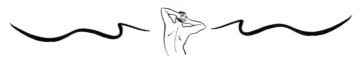

EXERCISE ~ PELVIC TILT

The pelvic tilt is a simple but very soothing exercise to do when your back is hurting. It's also a good way to learn proper alignment, so practise this exercise as often as you can.

The easiest way to learn a pelvic tilt is lying down. Once you get the hang of it, you can also practise it standing against a wall.

Lie with your feet flat on the floor, knees bent. Relax your arms by your side. Put one hand under the small of your back and feel the gap between that and the floor. Now press the small of your back into the floor and your hand by tightening your abdominal muscles and drawing your pubic bone upwards. Practise regularly until you can do this movement easily.

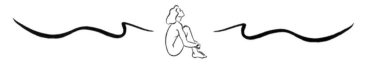

EXERCISE ~ ABDOMINAL WORK

Unless you consciously exercise them, your abdominal muscles may be very weak and will not offer any support to your back. Providing you exercise them in the right way, the abdominals respond very quickly to training, and will help protect your back. Toned abdominals, of course, also look attractive, so get practising.

Tips

- Coming up too far in a sit-up is ineffective as you are just working your hip flexors rather than your abdominals. It also puts your lower back under strain.

- Instead curl up slowly with control.

- Breathe out on exertion so that you flatten your stomach as you curl up.

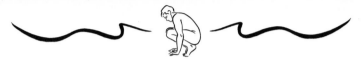

EXERCISE ~ ABDOMINAL WORK

- Don't worry if you can't come up more than a couple of inches off the floor at first. The important thing is that you feel the tension in your stomach.

- If your stomach muscles start to bunch you are coming up too far.

- You also strengthen your muscles on the way back down so do this slowly and with control. Don't just crash back to the floor.

- Sit up machines can be useful if you get neck ache as they keep your head and neck support. Otherwise just rest your hands gently behind your neck and let your stomach muscles do the work.

Classic Curl Up

Lie on the floor with your knees bent, feet flat on floor. Place your hands on your thighs. Slowly curl up. Pause. Curl back down. Pause

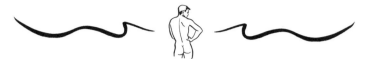

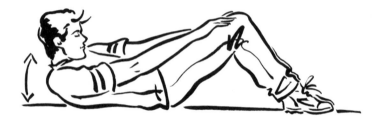

without resting on the floor in between reps. To focus on abdominal control try the curl ups with your forearms over your face, elbows together and fingers touching your forehead.

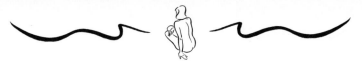

EXERCISE ~ ABDOMINAL WORK

Add A Twist

Start as in classic curl up. This time, rotate your shoulder so that you come up with one shoulder moving towards the opposite knee. You should feel the tension in the side of your stomach muscles (obliques). Once you've completed your reps, repeat on other side.

Reverse Curl

Lie on the floor, bending your knees and raising your feet in the air. This time you are initiating the curl from the other end of the spine. Slowly curl your bottom and lower back off the floor. Don't swing the legs as this will stop you using your stomach muscles as gravity will simply take over. The reverse curl is a very simple subtle movement that takes practice. Once you get the hang of it you can curl up from both

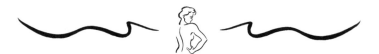

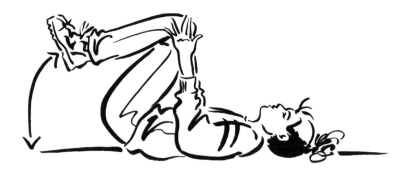

ends of the spine simultaneously (ie head, neck and shoulders curl up at the same time as lower back and bottom).

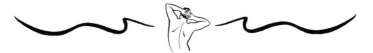

EXERCISE ~ ABDOMINAL WORK

Deep Core Muscles

The transverse abdominal muscles are located deep inside the stomach and are very important from a postural point of view. The easiest way to exercise these muscles is to simply suck your stomach in as though you are trying to create an inch or two of extra space within your waist band. Hold for a few seconds and then slowly release. Once you get used to retracting your stomach muscles in this way you can start to incorporate this into other exercises so that for example you suck your stomach in before even starting a curl up.

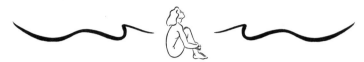

EXERCISE ~ SPORT

One of the biggest mistakes people make when suffering from back pain is giving up on sport altogether. Although certain back conditions need rest for a few days or even total rest, most back pain, particularly if it's muscular, will benefit from some activity.

Swimming is particularly kind and gentle to the back as your body weight is supported by the water. If you swim breast-stroke, make sure your spine stays well aligned and that you keep your neck long and face in the water when you're not coming up for air. Sports rehabilitation often takes place in water which can give a safe and surprisingly intensive workout.

Racquet Sports Certain sports such as racquet sports may aggravate

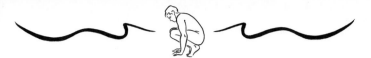

EXERCISE ~ SPORT

back pain as they encourage over-use of one side of the body. Make sure you balance this with some work on the other side. After a game of **tennis** or **squash**, for example, swing the racket a few times in your non-playing hand.

Yoga and **Pilates** are both particularly good for the back and can help prevent and alleviate back pain by encouraging good alignment. They will also improve your flexibility.

Sporting Tips

● In order to get the most out of your sport, you need to build up a good level of cardiovascular fitness. It's useful to keep a track of your heart rate as this shows if you're training hard enough. Your

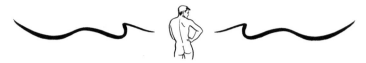

maximum heart rate can be calculated by subtracting your age from 220. For general fitness you should aim to train at 60-70% of your maximum heart rate. To boost your performance you should train to up to 80% of your maximum.

- After attaining a good level of general fitness, it's time to get sports specific. Stretch and strengthen the muscles you will be using in your chosen sport. There are many good books on this subject or it may be worth employing a personal trainer to devise a sports specific programme for you.

- If you do play sport, you have to expect that you may encounter the occasional mechanical problem. Most of these are usually self-regulating and you will be able to continue with your sport within a few weeks.

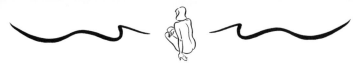

EXERCISE ~ SPORT

- Following an injury, return to low-impact activity, gradually building up repetition and weight.

- Sometimes a back injury means a change in sporting routine. As you get older you may need to choose something of lower impact.

- A cross-training approach is also much kinder to the back so that you vary your programme – ie walk one day, swim the next and run the day after. This helps avoid over-stressing any one part of the body.

- Buy appropriate footwear as this will reduce the load to the spine and joints.

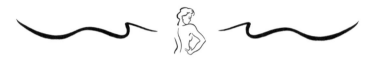

BACK TO LIFE

If you are suffering from a long-term or chronic back problem, the constant pain can easily get you down. Conventional medicine and alternative remedies can help.

In chronic cases, a visit to a pain psychologist can be very useful as he or she will teach you how to live with the problem in a positive way.

One of the worst things for chronic back pain sufferers is not the pain itself but all the other areas of their life it is affecting. Stresses such as how you are going to pay the mortgage, take the children to school, continue a sex life, can all add up to mental torture. Try to allow your life to get back to normal as much as possible. For example, if you've always loved running, but are scared to do it in case it aggravates the

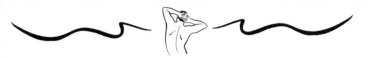

BACK TO LIFE

pain, check what your physical therapist thinks about this. It may be that running doesn't make the pain worse at all, in which case it's worth doing as it will do wonders for your self-esteem.

Above all, remember you're not alone. More than half the population are also suffering from back pain. Unfortunately, back pain is part of modern life. Instead of fighting, accept it. And try to make your life as healthy and enjoyable as possible.

Good luck. We hope this book has helped.

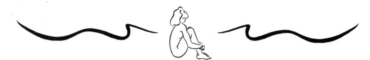

USEFUL CONTACTS

- National Back Pain Association~ 0181 977 5474

- General Osteopathic Council ~ 0171 357 6655

- British Acupuncture Council ~ 0181 964 0222

- British Chiropractic Association ~ 0118 950 5950

- Chartered Society of Physiotherapy ~ 0171 306 6666

- Pain Concern UK ~ 01227 712183

- Society of Teachers of the Alexander Technique (STAT)
  ~ 0171 351 0828

- Spinal Injuries Association
  ~ Counselling line 0181 833 4296 Mon-Fri 2-5pm

- The British Homoeopathic Association ~ 0171 935 2163

- National Institute of Medical Herbalists ~ 01392 426022